Change Weight Fast And Keep It Off Forever

Check out more articles and books by Chris Peters at www.theingeniouslifestyle.com

Reader Bonus

Thank you very much for buying my book! I deeply hope that this book, will help you change your mindset, optimize your eating habits and make you a better version of yourself.

As a small token of gratitude for my readers, I compiled a bonus report for you. You can use it as a guide, that will help you bring high-quality, clean food on your table. Here's the link to download your free report.

http://subscribe.theingeniouslifestyle.com/bonus

Table of Contents

Introduction

Thank you for choosing to read this book. It's been a labor of love for me and something I am really proud to share with you. It's a very important message I believe should be shared with as many people as possible because we have all dealt with the subject matter in some form or another.

I'm not going to bog you down with a lot of technical information and overload you with a ton of jargon that none of us really understands. I will keep my message simple but clear. If you're interested in more of the technical side of this topic, feel free to get online and do your own research. The purpose of this book is to give you clear and direct motivation about how to change your life.

My deepest passion is sharing the experiences I've learned with others. That includes you. I would love it if after reading this book it inspired you to go out there and be the biggest and best part of who you always wanted to be. This information has taken me years to learn and implement. That's due to all the time I wasted denying my situation. Hopefully, it won't take you that long. However, that's up to you. I can only do so much. I can give you the information, but it's absolutely useless unless you put it into action and do something about it.

The very first rule that I would love for you to grasp is that you are in control of your life. Nobody else. You are responsible for your actions and what you do or do not do. If you do not recognize that there's something in your life that needs to be changed, then there's no motivation to change it.

Take a long look at yourself and ask what is it that you need to improve. Admitting that you have shortcomings is the first step to getting on the road to building a better life. Nobody is going to ever love you as much as you should love yourself, so it's time to start giving that self-love.

And it doesn't have to start with some great big gesture. You can take baby steps. Set small, tiny goals, accomplish them, build your confidence and then set some more. Looking at the entire goal all at once is enough to scare anybody. It will only serve to paralyze you and put you into analysis paralysis where you will shut down and do absolutely nothing because it feels so overwhelming.

This book isn't about completely giving up everything you love. This is about a lifestyle transformation that is designed to last your entire life. That means that you are going to indulge in some of the foods that are not as good for you, but that you still love. The point is to gently incorporate healthier foods into your existing diet so that gradually you are moving to a healthier lifestyle, without going through a painful process.

Having said that, there will be some challenges. There's nothing you can do about it. In order to change some things, you're going have to endure the pain. But losing weight and getting healthy doesn't have to be one of them. We've been conned by the food and weight loss industry to believe that it is painful to change, but it really isn't. The industry has spent billions of dollars reaping the rewards of trying to convince you that you need to divert the pain of weight loss by buying their products.

The reality is that with the proper attitude and thinking, it isn't really painful (if you do it correctly). There is no cold turkey. There's no having to "white knuckle it" to endure the pain in order to get better. We're talking very small gradual changes, and adapting to one before starting on the others.

Your body is an amazing machine. Once it starts getting more of those healthier foods, it begins to crave them. This means it stops craving the bad foods. Your body will adapt to a lot of things and it will adapt to healthy food just as quickly as it does to junk food.

In fact, it's even more so the case because our bodies are designed to crave those things that mother nature grows in the wild for us to eat. Generations have lived for thousands of years based on these foods. It's only in recent times with the introduction to the Industrial Revolution that we have processed foods and chemicals laced in everything that we consume. This is why are having such a problem all over the world with the foods that we eat, and especially in this country.

Quick quote: *"Absorb what is useful for you discard what is useless and add what is specifically your own." - Bruce Lee*

Part 1
Challenge your Mindset

"Once your mindset changes, everything on the outside will change along with it."

Steve Maraboli, Life, the Truth, and Being Free

Chapter 1: My Story

I've been where you are now.

As a kid, I was fat and unhealthy throughout my entire childhood. I was miserable. Maybe you can relate, but it's a horrific feeling to be a kid and be constantly self-conscious about who you are. I can tell you that it does very little to help build self-esteem. Especially when mainstream society tells us what code of beauty should be. We must live by their rules, or be shunned.

I went to school and had other kids tease me because of what I looked like. It didn't matter who I was on the inside. Whether or not I was a good person with a loving and caring heart. None of that mattered. All everyone saw was the outside shell of a kid who was really unhappy.

This went on until I was 18 years old. Every day I would come home from school and shove Doritos and Coca-Cola into my stomach. Food was my only friend. That and watching television. I rarely went out and socialized.

And then one day I was watching the World Wrestling Entertainment channel. For the first time, I saw what I wanted to look like. Those men were in great shape with bulging biceps, awesome abs and a lot of confidence. I wanted to be like that, and at the same time, it made me feel so bad about my body because I didn't look like those wrestlers.

I knew that it must have taken a lot of work for those guys to get the muscles they had. I wanted to be in that good of shape. Something clicked in me. I realized that I wanted a better body more than I wanted to stay in my comfort zone surrounded by pizza, chips and sodas.

Being overweight had taken its toll on my body. I had no energy and could barely think straight because my brain felt foggy. I never wanted to go out into the world and do anything because I was embarrassed, but I was also exhausted all the time.

That all changed once I started learning how to eat healthier. I implemented several tiny changes. As a result, my mood went up and so did my energy levels. I was no longer lethargic.

Instead, I was motivated to get outdoors and do things. When I felt better I acted like I felt better. Meaning I went out and I did more things with more people. I participated in life which gave me the confidence to believe that I didn't have to be so self-conscious. I started to believe that I was a valued member of society who mattered.

The great thing was I realized I didn't have to spend a bunch of money on superfoods or buy all organic at those high-priced designer grocery stores. There were humble foods like spinach that became the main staple for me. There were inexpensive and very healthy options, both for my waistline and my budget.

So I'm telling you, if I can do this then you can do it. All it takes are baby steps and the willingness to put one foot in front of the other. As long as you never stop, you can never fail.

So let's get started.

Chapter 2: Do you really know what you buy when you go to the grocery store?

How do you shop? Do you plunk along one aisle to the next, picking up what looks good and hurling it into your cart? Do you shop when you're hungry? Do you go for the brightly colored packaging? For the promise of great taste?

There are so many choices that it gets confusing. In addition to that, manufacturers put special language on the boxes that tell you it's "healthy." Fat-free! No trans fat! Calorie-free! Sugar-free! The latest fad is automatically supposed to be healthy for you.

It's no wonder that we are suffering from major diseases and health problems because nobody knows who they can trust to tell them the truth.

Nobody understands which information is correct. GMO, for example. Do you know what that is? Do you know if it's in your food? What about other chemical artificial flavorings? Is it packed with salt and sugar? How many calories does it have? How many carbohydrates does it have?

If you don't have any idea as to what I'm talking about, that's okay. Most people don't. We mindlessly trust these big brand companies when they tell us that their food is good for us. We consume it because it tastes good. It triggers us to want more of it and then a vicious cycle begins. For example, a fruit salad could have the same calories as a can of Coke, but it depends on what's inside the ingredients of each. Fruit salad is packed with nutrients and fiber, while Coca-Cola is filled with sugar and artificial chemicals. So a calorie is a calorie is a calorie isn't necessarily true.

Do you want to know the crazy thing about all of this? We would never feed some of the stuff that we eat to our pets. It would be considered animal cruelty. We eat these ingredients because they are disguised with complex names that we don't take the time to research and find out what it really means. We just assume that the food industry (which is out to benefit from the billions we throw their way) are telling us the truth about what's in our food.

So, if you love your pets and you love your children, which I'm sure you do, why wouldn't you love yourself the same amount, if not more? You have to treat yourself well in order to be there for your family. Obviously, you don't want your children to become obese and unhealthy, so the same rules should apply to you.

You have to love yourself and your body so that you can enjoy it. Your mind and your body are only going to be able to run as efficiently as the fuel that you feed it. This is like taking a sports car and feeding it sand-laden gasoline and expecting it to run at peak performance. It doesn't happen. It breaks down and gets in all the gears. You've ruined the entire vehicle.

This is no different. And just because you don't always see the symptoms immediately, it does not mean that your body isn't slowly packing in the sludge that will definitely affect your health and well-being.

Chapter 3: "Begin with the end in mind."- *Stephen Covey's Seven Habits of Highly Effective People*.

Write down your eating habits and visualize how you will be if you eat like this for one month, one year, and 10+ years. Now do the same with healthy eating habits.

Don't skip over this part. Mindset is key and if you can visualize it clearly in your head then you will be able to achieve it. Did you know that your brain can't tell the difference between your dreams and your reality? It will act "as if" on anything that you think about. So that's why mindset training really works because if you visualize it and act as if what you want has already happened then your mind will assume it is real. That's the first step to getting what you want.

So take the time to do the visualization exercise. Do you see any difference? Which one feels better to you? Is that cake or fast food that you're about to eat worth it?

Quick tip: Next time you are about to eat something, make sure to acknowledge if this food serves your body and your purpose. Or is it just a short-term enjoyment that will eventually backfire?

Chapter 4: *"There are no facts, only interpretations"* - Friedrich Nietzsche.

Nothing is going to happen to you until you decide it. That means you have to change your attitude and you have to have the willingness to do it. Nobody else can do this for you. You come into this earth and you go out of this earth as one being. You have the free will to make the choices on what to do in between that time.

Your attitude is going to dictate how successful you're going to be with this. If something sounds painful, you need to change the language in your head. Make your brain understand it in a better, more positive light.

For example, you're not dieting. You're transforming your lifestyle to accommodate a healthier active you who gets out, does things and is popular with their friends and in their community. Be the person you always wanted to be.

In order to do that, it means feeding your body the right fuel. Put another way, think about every single piece of junk food that you eat. Is it based on emotional eating? Fear? Anger? Why are you eating that? Are you even hungry? Is it the first thing you grabbed? Is it easier than cooking? What does that say about your thinking? Are you willing to settle for instant gratification rather than getting up, going to the refrigerator and getting something healthier?

Your daily actions determine the kind of person you are. Does it match with the person you always wanted to be? That's who you want to be when you're thinking about your eating.

Having said that, this is a process, not a sprint. So, let's say you drink coffee with sugar in it every day. I am not advising you to cut cold turkey. What I am saying is make a conscious decision every day to measure out your sugar and then decrease it in equal amounts each day so that you slowly wean yourself off. Get used to the way it tastes with healthier options. This doesn't have to happen overnight, but you have to be progressively moving forward.

In other words, you need to track this and not just eyeball it. You need to know how your progress is moving along on a daily basis and what you're doing toward your goal. This builds your self-esteem and as a result, you will build more confidence each day knowing that you are completing steps to become the person you always wanted to be.

Many new age diseases come from bad eating habits. So why do you think that within the last hundred years diseases, obesity, and cancer have all risen, compared to the last thousand? Could it be because of all the chemicals that are being put into our foods to preserve it, giving it a longer lifespan so that companies can make more money selling it?

And of course, more health problems mean more medical expenses, which of course you have to go to a doctor to get any kind treatment for where they essentially hold the treatments hostage for you to pay it or have insurance that can pay it.

My point is that if you neglect healthy eating, you essentially neglect your health which puts you at serious risk of shaving off a considerable number of years of your lifespan. On the other hand, by getting clean and nutritious food to help your immune system, you greatly reduce the possibilities of having serious diseases in the future.

I realize nobody ever wants to think about this, especially when we're young because the effects aren't always immediate. We often put it in the back of our minds and deny that anything will happen to us. We just go on continue eating the way we want and not getting enough exercise in our lifestyle.

Wouldn't it be amazing to be able to eat the same foods even when you are 50, 60 or 70+ years old? Wouldn't it be amazing to have a higher quality of life where you will enjoy every moment to its fullest? Eating healthy is a perfect beginning for that and I totally understand that it may seem difficult or overwhelming, but a journey of 1000 miles starts with one step. Let's do this together.

Quick reflection: *Think about this. Imagine you are 50 years old, and your doctor has diagnosed you with heart disease because of a lifetime of bad eating habits and inactivity. Visualize how you would feel hearing this news. Would you automatically wonder how much time you have left? Would you feel sorrow for missing your loved ones and wishing that you could have done something differently?*

You have that time right now. You have that opportunity. You have the ability to have a wake-up call to make a change. And for those of us who take that opportunity, we don't want to wait or push it out of our minds or deny that are spiraling downward.

We can make a change and not only extend our lifespan but also give it more quality and value.

And for those that argue that you could die any day, so you might as well live how you want, that's true. However, what if nothing does happen to you, as is actually the case for the vast majority of the people? What if your lifespan is solely dependent upon your physical health? Wouldn't you rather prepare for that scenario?

Chapter 5: Why Inuit and other traditional tribes did not have health problems.

Without being a historian, let me think about this right off the top of my head. Traditional tribes don't go to fast food restaurants. They don't go to McDonald's or Pizza Hut. They find their food from the land and they burn a ton of calories trying to find that food every single day.

Meanwhile, we can drive to the nearest restaurant and order anything we want off the "extra value menu," eat more calories in one sitting than we should have in a day, and then wait until two or three hours later when we do it all over again. At least three times a day.

We've spent a ton of money on junk food to fill a particular kind of need and most the time that need isn't even hunger. Then, we don't initiate any kind of consistent exercise program because most of us have jobs that are sedentary.

These tribes have a clean diet. By default, they don't have a choice and as a result, they live healthier lifestyles. I realize it's hard because we do have choices. We have a lot of choices, but we are still responsible for our own self-discipline to say no to those things that would harm us.

A diet is made to serve you as a guideline. Use your own intuition when needed and don't become a slave to the concept of a diet. Watch what you eat and balance it with happiness and healthy options. It's perfectly fine to be a foodie, but a foodie knows that they eat responsibly for taste and experience, not hoarding and gluttony.

Chapter 6: The real reason that you get cravings and how to start changing your mindset.

The following summation of how our brains interact with food will shed a lot of light as to why we keep craving for. High-fat and especially high sugar foods are high energy, which is exactly why we feel cravings for them. They are like gold for our animal brains, which are programmed to consume as many high-energy foods as possible for survival purposes. When our ancestors foraged or hunted for their meals, sugar was quite rare; this is why they signaled our brains with a huge endorphin release - the chemical of anticipation and desire. Because they were so rarely found in nature, there was no need for a protective mechanism against overconsumption. We were supposed to consume them whenever we were lucky enough to stumble upon them. The problem is that the "food revolution" happened extremely fast, evolutionary speaking. Within a century we could have any food within arm's reach but our brains did not have the time to evolve into this type of scenario.

So when you eat that delicious candy, you get this amazing endorphin release and you crave for more. It's almost as addictive as being on drugs. But the nutrients, fibers and minerals that your body desperately need are not there, and that is the main source of our problems.

Another challenge we have is that while eating clean is most of the secret, you also need to get into an exercise lifestyle to keep your health up and weight down. Toxins from the food we eat, build up in our bodies if we don't keep our bodies fit and exercise. That's when all the problems start.

I've said it before and I'm probably going to say it again. You need to take small manageable steps. Do not ever beat yourself up for sliding back and eating something that you shouldn't. In fact, you should be eating some of those foods if that's what you normally eat and incorporating healthy foods on the side until eventually, you transform into eating mostly healthy foods with a side of something that's not as healthy.

Don't over think it right now. Continue doing what you're doing, only add healthy options at each meal. Pretty soon it will become a habit and you won't even think about it.

Part 2

Know Your Food

"Tell me what you eat, and I will tell you what you are."

Anthelme Brillat-Savarin

Chapter 7: Organic or not?

The food industry has gotten so bad that it's getting to the point where we can't even find healthy organic foods anymore. And if we do, it's astronomically expensive. However, some companies are getting competitive and grocery stores are starting to provide organic options.

That doesn't mean you can blindly trust what they're telling you. You still need to read the label. Sometimes unscrupulous companies claim an item is organic when in fact, it is not. They use deceptive language to make you think it is healthier than it is. When in fact, it may not be the case.

Educating yourself about what's on the label and how to read it is very important. You want to be a conscientious consumer. The ideal scenario is to endeavor to have 100% organic food that's grown clean, processed, and harvested. For example, if you eat fast food two or more times a week, then start choosing healthier items on the menu.

This is what I mean about small changes. Get a salad or remove the bun on a burger. Try something different that leads you closer to your ultimate goal of creating a new habit to replace the bad one.

Chapter 8: Vegan or not?

The good news is, this book isn't about one side or the other. You can be vegan, vegetarian or a meat eater. I'm not going to debate the virtues of each. This is all about implementing a healthy lifestyle that will make you feel good, live longer and help you be disease-free.

It's true that in our society it is very difficult to find free range chickens and grass fed animals and when you do, it tends to be on the more expensive side. It's easy to eat clean if you have a plant-based diet, but I want to stress that you can do both.

When eating clean becomes second nature, then you can move to grass-fed, free-range animals products and more organic-based items. This is the ideal, but you can work up to it and still see results in improved health and weight loss. The biggest, most important point is not to overwhelm yourself.

Chapter 9: What about checking the nutrition label?

Checking how many calories each food has is going to make you crazy and overwhelm you, if you don't know how to do it correctly. You need to know how to check the nutritional data and be able to differentiate good from bad calories, carbohydrates, fats, protein, sugar, salt, etc.

The main goal is to find good, clean food.

Quick tip: The more ingredients a food has, the more processed it usually is.

Here's a great piece of knowledge you should hold on to when in a grocery store. Everything that is against the walls on the outer perimeter of the store is usually a healthier food option. That's where you're going to find the meats, fruits and vegetables.

Everything in the middle or center of the grocery store you want to try to stay away from. It's mostly all processed food. If it has a brief shelf life, chances are it's going to be healthier for you, since it might contain fewer conservatives. The excellent thing about this is that you can eat a lot more of these kinds of foods - fruits and vegetables. For example, have you ever known anyone to become obese from eating too much broccoli?

Quick tip: Once you start eating clean, you will see a big difference in your mood and your tolerance to process unhealthy foods. After eating healthy for a while your own body will lower its tolerance to processed and junk food. Even your taste will improve and your tongue receptors will begin to be more sensitive to any kind of taste.

Chapter 10: What differentiates healthy food from unhealthy food?

In order to answer this question, we have to define the word healthy. What does healthy mean to you? Maybe you think this question is ridiculous. After all, everybody knows what healthy means, right?

The problem is usually they don't because otherwise, the health and food industries would not be worth billions of dollars like they do now. They get their profits by convincing you that one thing is healthy, while another thing is not. Then the next month, something else is deemed healthy. New fad diets or methods to lose weight are on a carousel, constantly being traded in and out for the latest, greatest shiny object.

Doctors aren't much better because nobody can give you a straight answer. There's so much bad information out there. So much noise that keeps us from understanding how to live a basic healthy lifestyle. It also depends on who you listen to because one group may stress to only eat things that are alive and then another group will say the opposite.

Let's talk about calories.

How many calories does a person need? A sedentary person may need 2,500 calories or even less. A bodybuilder might eat 4,000 calories per day intentionally "carb loading" when trying to add muscle mass, but for someone who isn't a bodybuilder, that's probably not the best measuring stick for them. There are so many variables (weight, metabolism, exercise etc.) which shape our daily caloric intake. Trying to keep track of it during the day is usually a very painful and frustrating process. When we stick to calories, we tend to become a slave of the system and also forget to actually enjoy our food. The caloric food ratio is meant to serve us, not vice versa. Don't get me wrong. I highly appreciate the value of this system because it is scientific and very accurate. However, for a normal person like ourselves, it's better to find an easier, more efficient way to differentiate healthy from unhealthy food.

So, in order to determine the definition of healthy you have to ask a different question. Ask yourself which foods cause chronic disease and obesity and which foods are less likely to do that. This is a better place to start. Then as time goes by and you feel comfortable, if you want you can learn more about calories. Baby stepping is the key!

Chapter 11: Interesting facts about healthy eating that will absolutely blow your mind.

Eighty percent of what is sold in local supermarkets has added sugar in it. I mean, that might seem like just another number until you take a second and really think about what 80% looks like. That means that only 20% of what is sold in the supermarket might be in its original form. Only a fifth!

This totally blew me away and I really started to adjust my thinking on a number of useless products on the market that really don't offer much nutritional value.

Next, when you are talking about sugar content, usually there is no difference between full-fat and low-fat products. They can both contain the exact same amount of it, and the same applies for additives and preservatives. Furthermore, the low-fat choices are even more processed and tend to have extra additives or chemicals, in order to achieve the same texture as the full-fat product. Next time you choose to go for the low-fat, light product, that claims to be a healthier choice, make sure to double-check the ingredients.

Quick exercise: Pick up two products and make a quick comparison between the full-fat product and the low-fat one. First, check the sugar content, then check if they have the same ingredients. Are they the same? A very good example is mayonnaise. The lighter it gets the more ingredients it usually has.

I am a very strong supporter of the farmer's market, as I believe it's worth it to pay a little more for quality food. However, I noticed these days that a lot of the companies are trying to market some of their sugary preservative-filled products as being organic.

Apparently, the FDA allows it so that you can get away with labeling a product organic. If there is one ingredient in the product that is in fact organic approved, the entire product can be approved.

They use clever phrases like "made with organic ingredients" or "gluten-free" when it's not even a wheat product. For instance, at certain fast food joints, they often say "this contains 100% Alberta beef". This is a cleverly phrased statement because it's true that the *beef part* in the patty is indeed 100% Alberta beef, but what it fails to say is that usually, just a tiny fraction of the actual patty consists of beef. The rest are MSG additives and chemicals that they add for taste enhancement as well as a good percentage of filler, which is far less appealing than the perceived 100% beef patty.

According to a research published in the US National Library of Medicine *"amongst the eight fast food hamburger patties tested, meat content ranged between 2.1 and 14.8 percent, with an average of about 12.1 percent."*

But people read that statement as my burger is 100% Alberta beef and therefore a healthy source of iron, but sadly that's not the case.

Chapter 12: What is processed food?

Processed foods are the opposite of naturally grown foods. Basically, processed describes how the food is put together from the time it was created, to the moment it hits your plate. Many times processed food is anything with more than one ingredient. The more work that is required to get it in an edible condition, the fewer nutrients and minerals are left in it. This means you can develop a severe lack of proper vitamins in your body and the risk of malnutrition.

Even though you're eating a lot of processed foods you are not getting the vitamins and minerals you need to sustain your body's healthy function. Having said all that, some organic foods could be processed as well. For example, wheat, lean meats, vegetables and fruits; they can all be put through processing that makes them edible. Processing can include steaming, grinding, chopping, extensive heat, canning and preserving it in sugar or salt. The best idea is for you to stick to unprocessed foods that are organically grown and are the closest to their natural state.

Main points to consider:

- *Healthy food is not necessarily more expensive.* You just have to find the right deal.
- *Know what you're looking for.*
- *Make sure that what you're paying for is what you're getting.*
- *The food industry can be very tricky.* Some "healthy" food will try to mimic all the taste choices as junk food. They do make Oreos that are an organic, or minimally processed option. That doesn't mean it's completely healthy and you should eat five packs of them. It means that is a better option than the traditional junk food.
- *Healthy food does not take longer to prepare.* That's a common misconception. You can find hundreds of recipes that take less than 30 minutes to prepare. Once you get started and get into the right mindset, you will prepare sexy looking, healthy food in no time.
- *Healthy eating does not mean having to deny yourself.* On the contrary, eating healthy foods allows you to eat more. I guarantee that you're going to get full faster before you have the opportunity eat as much as you could eat with junk.

Part 3
Take Action

"Don't let your learning lead to knowledge. Let your learning lead to action."

Jim Rohn

Chapter 13: 10 hacks to lose weight fast and keep it off forever

Hack 1: Decrease your sugar intake

It's delicious.

It's tasty.

And the more of you eat, the more you can't get enough of it. It's our good pal sugar. The temptress of taste buds found in everything we eat. Nowadays it's nearly impossible to find anything in the grocery store that doesn't contain some amount of sugar in it. From condiments like ketchup and barbecue sauce to sugary cereal. Sugar is everywhere.

If there's only one thing you learn from this book, it's this: Decrease the amount of sugar from your diet. Try to get it out of your daily consumption is much as possible. If you can't, then at least minimize the amount to eventually wean yourself off of it. Sugar is a killer. It will slowly destroy your body which is why it's important that you keep track of the ingredients in the food that you eat.

Sugar wreaks havoc on your body, causing your insulin to spike. You can throw your body into shock so you want to avoid all foods that are high in sugar and that includes condiments and those things that are not readily expected to be in sugar like ketchup. Don't rip out all the sugar all at once because your body will go into terrible withdraws. The last thing you want is to deal with headaches and flu-like symptoms.

Purposefully limit each day how much additional sugar you take in. Each day (or take it a week at a time) decrease it a little bit until you get to the point where doesn't bother you. The secret here is to keep your meals balanced. That means an equal amount of carbs, proteins and healthy fats at each meal. The fat serves to satiate those cravings for sweet and salty things.

Make sure you're eating four to six small meals a day, every two to three hours. This keeps your metabolism going, and the reason for that is that our bodies are made to survive. This is especially true when there's a shortage of food.

We adapt by our metabolism slowing down and going into survival mode, thereby storing as much fat as it possibly can to keep us alive. Eating once a day tells your body exactly that, "burn the least you can - food is scarce".

Only eating once or twice a day, gives your body the starvation signal so it does what it knows how to do and it starts holding on to everything it has. So if you want to lose weight and get healthier, then you need to eat more often (not more food!). Eating four to six times a day allows your body to get all the nutrients and minerals it needs. It will signal to your body that it can let go of the extra fat because it realizes more is coming. Eating smaller, more frequent meals will keep your blood sugar level stable.

So stay away from processed foods and try to stick to the outlying areas of the grocery stores I mentioned earlier. Try to get fruits and vegetables and lean meats in your system. Pre-planning is the secret to doing this. Even if you have to cook your food for the week on a Sunday, it makes it a lot easier for you to stick with this type of lifestyle.

Salt is also another ingredient that should be limited. Too much salt is not good for you. Try Himalayan salt as an alternative to regular salt. Make sure it's actual Himalayan salt since some producers add pink food coloring to regular salt and market it as Himalayan.

Hack 2: Be wise when it comes to fats

We need a certain amount of good fat to keep our bodies in good working order. Coconut oil and olive oil are two examples of good fats that help keep your body healthy. If you want butter or dairy products, make sure that they are grass fed and range free. Otherwise, if the animals consume grain, you are ultimately eating grain.

Does that make you fat? Not necessarily. It depends on the kind of fat that you're eating. You want to avoid trans fats and stick to any good fats like coconut oil and olive oil, which have great health benefits. Grass fed butter is the better option than processed butter and especially margarine. Don't eat margarine. Did you know that margarine is one molecule away from plastic? It's very bad for you. So bad in fact that you'll never see flies buzzing around it.

Quick tip: Eating fat does not make you fat. You can eat butter every day and still be lean and healthy. The whole concept is to realize how much fat your body actually needs and keep it there. The average recommended fat intake for males is about 70gr/day and 50gr for females. To give you a quick idea 100gr of cheese usually have around 30gr of fat and one tablespoon of butter has approximately 12-14gr.

Hack 3: Eat slowly and mindfully

Balance your meals each time you eat and keep your portions modest. It takes your stomach about 20 minutes to get the message from your brain that you're not hungry anymore. But until that time, if you keep eating, you're going to take on more calories, carbs and fats than you need.

Our portion sizes have gotten out of control because we've stopped paying attention to our food. Now we eat in front of the television or while we're on the go and we don't stop to enjoy it or to even realize what we just ate. It's important to do nothing else but eat your food when it's time. Turn off all distractions and concentrate on the intention of chewing, tasting and swallowing.

When you have to eat at a restaurant or fast food place, don't automatically "super size" your meal. You don't need all the unnecessary added fat, calories, salt and cholesterol that comes with value meals. Treat your body right by eating slowly and enjoying your food. It will keep you fuller longer and give your brain the message that you are satisfied.

You can actually eat just about everything that you want to eat as long as you keep the quantity portion size normal. Overdoing it is where we run into trouble. Balance in everything you do including your meals. Listen to your body and eat only when it tells you that it's hungry.

Hack 4: Listen to your body

For example, if you're going to the gym and working out for a very long time you want to increase the amount of food you eat. It's all relative and should be balanced with common sense and education. Instead of eating candy, try dried fruit. Yes, there's still sugar in there but it's a different type of sugar and a step in a healthier direction. Remember this is a lifestyle transformation. It does not and should not happen in one day. It's going to take some time, but as long as you keep moving forward you can't fail. Try to limit fruit juices as they contain a large amount of sugar. Eat the real thing instead. It has the fiber you need to keep your system cleaned out and healthy.

You want to preplan your meals so that you have good foods instead of reaching for something that isn't good for your body.

Instead of sweets, try nuts. They have great nutritional value and the right fats that you need. Introduce a little bit when you're snacking, and you'll soon realize that you're getting used to it a lot faster than you thought you could.

When you try to bake or use ingredients, you can substitute organic versions of flour and butter. All you have to do is look for them in the right section. A lot of organic sections are now popping up in grocery stores, or you can go to the grocery stores that are specifically targeted toward whole foods.

Quick tip: The more nutrient dense and less processed food you eat, the fuller you will feel. You won't care about the quantity because you will naturally eat less.

Take carrots, for example. They're so nutritious and fulfilling that you can eat as much as you want without worrying about how it will negatively impact your body. These healthy foods are more fulfilling and will actually make you feel fuller than its counterpart. Choose nutrient dense foods.

This is important enough to say it again:

When you're talking about juice, make sure you keep the pulp in there. Juicing strains out all the good fiber and nutrients in the fruit leaving you with sugary juice that can spike insulin levels. It's better to make smoothies. Not to mention you throw away most of the fruits and vegetables. That's an unnecessary waste of money.

There's the instant gratification mindset and then there's the patience mindset where you lie in wait for what you really want.

Which personality type are you?

Many of us are instant gratification personalities because that's what our society has become. Everything is available at the tip of our fingertips. At the drop of a hat, or with one phone call, anything we've ever wanted, we can now have relatively easily. This includes food, which is why you want to be very mindful of what you're eating and not settle into the habit of mindlessly snacking when you should be eating healthier options.

Like I said, pay attention to your food. Don't eat while you're watching TV or doing something else. Concentrate solely on the food that you're eating because focusing on it makes it a conscious act and will prevent you from overeating.

Hack 5: Enjoy a good breakfast

When you eat breakfast you're going to boost your metabolism and keep your sugar levels stable in order to avoid overwhelming cravings throughout the day. Even if you don't want to eat breakfast, try to eat anyway because it really does start your day out on the right foot. It's much better to eat a small breakfast over nothing at all. You have to start your metabolism in the morning so breakfast is a must.

Quick tip: Drink water and eat some bread with olive oil about half hour before you actually eat. This will help you control your appetite and help you eat the right amount of food. Whole-grain is the purest, most unprocessed grain, so it's always a better choice.

Hack 6: Freeze it up and pick seasonal products

If you can't buy fresh fruits and vegetables, frozen is the next best thing. It's very convenient to use and if you freeze it properly, you can keep it intact with its nutritional value.

Find food that's in-season

Usually, foods at the farmers market are unprocessed, fresher and very inexpensive. Not to mention it's obviously better for you. Keep in mind that you are baby stepping your way to a healthier transformation and lifestyle.

When you go to the grocery store, substitute one or two processed foods for more natural options. Then gradually increase it by one more until eventually, you're only buying healthy food that's good for you and maybe the occasional snack.

Here's a quick guide to give you an idea about seasonal foods!

http://theingeniouslifestyle.com/seasonal-food-list/

Hack 7: Plan Ahead

Plan ahead of time by cooking your food. It's best to prepare and package your meals so that all you have to do is open the refrigerator and grab one perfectly proportioned meal.

Quick tip: Eating salads? There are tons of DIY salad dressings you can make yourself that contain only the best ingredients. Take a few minutes and do this. It will keep you on track. It's hard sometimes to realize how much salad dressing we're eating, but if you really stopped and looked at it, it's way more than what we need with all that sugar and salt packed inside.

Hack 8: Beware of Drinking Calories

Be careful of drinking your calories, especially in sodas and alcohol. This is a vital factor to consider when you work your way into a healthier lifestyle. It doesn't seem like it at all, but in a very short time you can put on a lot of weight because of what you're drinking. Alcoholic drinks are loaded with empty calories (no nutritional value) and usually contain many carbohydrates and added sugar. Did you know that drinking a Mojito or two glasses of whiskey, will give you the same calories as eating one regular portion of roasted chicken breast? Or the same as eating a ham & cheese sandwich? Not to mention that it's bad for your kidneys and liver, which have to work overtime to filter out those toxins.

Hack 9: Cut Your Portion Sizes

Cut your portion sizes down so that you're not eating supersized portions. The fast food industry has made a killing from promoting the concept that more is better. Eating a big fat supersized value meal has enough calories, fat and carbohydrates to feed three people, literally. Make sure that the fruits and vegetables that you are eating are taken from several different parts of the rainbow. This ensures you are getting a variety of minerals and nutrients to your body. Grass-fed and free range animals are the best type of meat to eat. Avoid animals who are being fed hormones, grain, corn or any other processed food. The same goes for chickens. If you're eating eggs, make sure that they are free-range.

Hack 10: Do not Bring it in the House

A great way to avoid eating bad food is not bringing in your house. This is the part that's going to require a certain amount of purposeful thought and self-control. Make sure that you do not start a habit of bringing in chips or candy or things that you know aren't good for your body. It's not worth it to feel so bad.

Instead, use spices and herbs to improve the taste of chicken and other meats so that you can add flavor and enjoy your food much better without relying on sugar and carbohydrates to the job for you.

Quick tip: Many tribes over the years used herbs and spices as medicine or to prevent diseases.

I totally agree that Western medicine has saved millions of lives, especially when we consider serious threatening diseases, but with clean and healthy eating we can either prevent many of these diseases before they even appear. Many herbs and spices have extraordinary healing and curing abilities. I would love to cover all these in another book because herbs and spices have helped me a lot.

Part 4

Commit To Your New Lifestyle

"Commitment is what transforms a promise into reality"

Abraham Lincoln

Chapter 14: Do You Have Your Mind Right?

Do you ever wonder why some people can keep their weight under control? Does it make you nuts trying to work it out in your head just what it is that they do that you're not doing? Do you feel a pang of envy because it seems so effortless for them? Great body, great skin, great life.

They're lucky, right? Wrong.

Chances are they work for the body they have. They commit hours, days, years to improving their health. They sacrifice other things in life to have their fitness.

Of course, there are people who simply have the genetics to eat as much as they want and not gain a pound, but even then as they age it tends to catch up with them. Regardless of weight gain or loss, health and fitness are still relevant to every human regardless of size.

Are you willing to give up as much to get what YOU want?
Are you even sure you want what they have? Or are you pursuing it because you think it's going to make you happy? Fill up that one spot in your life that's lacking?
Who do you live for?
Your parents? Your spouse? Children? Friends and family?
We all start out with the same 24 hours in each day but know this.
Regardless of what you achieve, it won't mean a hill of beans if you aren't committed to following through with it.
And being focused on what someone else is doing is taking focus on what you should be doing which is improving your own life.
You've got to get your mind right.
That means stop worrying about what other people are going to think about your choices.
Stop pursuing those things that don't satisfy you.

Take back your life. Simplify it and chase only those things that make you truly happy. Being healthy and fit is the center of everything else. It is the foundation upon which your life is built around.

No health, no life.

But I can tell you this all day long. It doesn't matter who gives you great advice if you aren't open to hearing it and taking action.

That's what you have to decide.

How bad do you want it?

Each day we wake up and are confronted with options.

We can do those things that are easy, the things we want to do.

OR

We can do those things that must be done in order to give us those things we truly desire.

Marginal happiness or pure blissful transformational happiness.

It's your choice.

Doesn't' seem so hard when you spell it out, does it? But you and I know that it actually is hard to put ourselves first. We love those who are in our lives and we put their needs ahead of our own while we woefully neglect ourselves.

You and I can't do that forever.

Don't you think you DESERVE to be proud of yourself?

Of course, you do. You deserve the undying happiness waiting on the other side of what it takes to go out and get it.

It can be hard at times. I get it and know firsthand how it feels.

Perhaps you don't want to workout every day.

Perhaps it's too difficult.

Perhaps it's painful and the experience isn't something you want to repeat daily.

And perhaps you don't feel you even deserve great health.

But let's get real here. If you can't do what it takes to get healthier, then you will NEVER be successful in losing weight and feeling better. So it's not really a choice. YOU have to come first. Your needs must be met before all others so you can take care of those you love.

When I was just starting my fitness journey, I remember how hard it was. I had to make the same decision to take action every single day.

Every time I wanted to stop healthy eating I had to make a choice. And every time I didn't want to go to the gym, I had to make a choice.

I spent years believing that I couldn't have the body I wanted. It was possible for others, but not an option for me.

Until one day when it all clicked and I began asking myself different questions. Why couldn't I do what others were doing and getting similar results?

It took choosing to do the work each and every day for me to gain the momentum to keep going.

Now I realize why all my past attempts at losing weight never worked. I wasn't committed. I didn't ask my brain the right questions. I didn't want it bad enough each and every day.

I found success because I made the decision to be open to being successful and then did the work every day to fulfill my dream into a reality.

And you are no different.

You can do the exact same thing. It's all about your mindset and what you choose to believe.

What are you going to believe?

Chapter 15: So What's Next?

No matter what you choose to do in the future about your health, make a conscious decision that you will not make yourself feel bad about where you are now. Being hard on yourself isn't just bad for your confidence, it's a futile attempt and wasted energy. There's nothing you can do about the past, except to leave it in the past.

Instead get excited about the present and the future. Get excited about the fact that this very second you have the power to choose your destiny. You decide which direction the next step you take is going to lead you. Which way will you go?

Will you continue to follow the same patterns as yesterday? Or will you try something new and different? If you continue to do what you've always done and expect a different result, you are just setting yourself up for failure and frustration.

I've been there and it's no fun.

In fact, it's torture. And it leads to nothing but more self-loathing and procrastination.

More of sitting on the couch wasting the hours watching television about worlds that you aren't going out and living.

More of feeling like you have to apologize to everyone for who you are and the way you look.

More of not being the ideal you that you always promised yourself you would be.

You are far too brilliant to settle for ordinary- aren't you?

Yes, you are.

You are a warrior. You have what it takes to change your life. And it doesn't have to be a superhero costume change with action words like POW! BANG! ZOOM! to change.

You can do it by taking a million baby steps each day. Each one moving you closer to your destiny. The place where you always wanted to be.

You know that place.

It's the one you dreamed of as a child. The absolute space in time where you are forever happy.

Because you became your own hero. You did what you needed to do to fulfill who you needed to be.

And all it took was to take that first step.

It can be hard. It can be the hardest thing you ever do in your life. But it can also be the most important step you ever take.

So what's stopping you?

Ah…

I know what it is.

It's the same demon that haunts us all.

It hunts down our happiness and slaughters it before we even get a chance to gasp our last breath.

Fear.

Who knew that four little letters could contain a whole lotta scary. But it's there. Every single day. Hiding in the shadows just daring us to think that we could possibly do something good with our lives.

Step outside of our comfort zones.

Break some rules.

Ride with the top down and our hands in the air.

Nope. Fear doesn't let us do any of that. It threatens us with a mean look like our mamma used to give us when we were about to do something we knew we shouldn't be doing.

It stands in the way with it's best friend and fellow bully "pain," and together they threatened a good old fashioned beating if we even so much as dared to dream that anything we wanted was possible.

But what if?

What if, instead of doing what you've always done, which is hesitate to the point of inaction, try something different. Stop thinking so much and start taking action to trust your first instinct to know that you need to do what has to be done.

Instead of allowing fear to control you by worrying that you're going to fail yet again, turn your brain off, trust your gut and do what you have to do. Stop spending your life complaining about what you don't like and start using the rest of your life to do something about it.

Don't you see? That's the only thing in this world that really truly matters. Confronting those fears and debunking them. Trust what your insides are telling you and listen to them. Stop at nothing to do whatever is necessary to get you to your goal. If that means eating healthier and working out more then that's what it means. Because so far you've tried it your way and it doesn't work, right?

So maybe it's time to try something different. If you continue to allow yourself to settle into the comfortable fear that you've been in nothing will ever change and everything that you feared is going to come true. Because you're going to create exactly what you fear. Your brain is a machine and if you ask it a question, it will give you an answer. That's why negative self-talk is so damaging to your self-esteem.

Have your negative fears gotten you to where you are right now? Once you start asking your brain the right questions you're going to get better answers and results.

But first, you have to get clear on what it is that you want. Do you want to get healthier? Do you want to lose weight? Do you want to feel better? Anything you want to do can happen as soon as you are very clear about what you want to change. It can be as fast as the blink of an eye.

But if you don't conquer that fear. It's going to stop you every single time. Look, it's impossible not to feel fear because that's part of our survival mechanism. Fear can save us from hurting ourselves in this world, but fear should be channeled and tempered with good judgment and a certain amount of risk-taking.

But you can't allow it to control you. You can no longer allow it to rule your life, invade your home and your family and hold you hostage. It will tear down every bit of self-esteem and confidence you have. It will create a monster with those you love and put a dividing wall between yourself and the outside world. If you want to be healthy. There is no way around it, you must first conquer fear and do the things that you don't want to do.

You're here right now because you want something different.

You're here because you're tired of doing it the same way and getting no or terrible results.

You're here because you want somebody to give you permission to step outside of yourself and do things differently.

I give you permission to be great. To succeed. To throw your fears to the side and act bravely. There's only one way over that cliff and that is to jump wholeheartedly with both feet. All in and no regrets. And when you do? Amazing things start to happen. Your thinking begins to shift. Your reality alters to include this new normal. When you stop white knuckling it is when you're going to start seeing results.

Step outside of this comfort zone of yours and dare to reach for something greater than yourself. No matter what happens you will surprise yourself. You will learn that you are braver, stronger than you thought you could be.

This leads to unbelievable internal dialogue that tells you-you can accomplish anything. That nothing is out of your reach. It is only a matter of you deciding that you want to be better and healthier.

When I was willing to change my patterns in my lifestyle. That's when it happened. One day motivated me to the next day and that's what kept me going. I took it day-by-day.

But you have to demand it from yourself. You have to tell yourself that you want these kinds of results. You want to feel healthier, lose weight, feel better. You are the only one who can lay down the law with yourself and declare that you will no longer tolerate less than what you know you can be. You can ask yourself what you need to do and who you need to be in order to get the results you're looking for. And the only thing that's left? Is to do what it takes to get that result. You'll be blown away by how fast you'll get results when you stop thinking so much about it and you start doing something about it.

In order to do that, you need to assume the sale. That means you need to assume that you already have that desired result. And then you're going to walk around and act as if it already belongs to you.

That's why I knew that I could get healthy because as soon as I committed to being that best part of myself. I acted as if it already happened. And every day my mind reaffirmed the fact that I knew I was already there.

You don't need anybody's permission to do this. You don't need positive affirmations from friends and family to tell you it's okay to get started. There are no false starts. Every day is an opportunity to move forward. You will be shocked at how fast you'll get results if you stop thinking so much about it and you start doing what it takes.

Are you willing to do what it takes?

I certainly hope so and I wish you all the best.

Chapter 16: Thank you

I would like to personally thank you for reading this book. We put a lot of effort to compile it and our main goal is to provide value to your lives.

I deeply wish that this book gave you the spark to become a better, healthier version of yourself. You are capable of anything! As they say, impossible is nothing. So the best time to act is now!

It is far better to take small imperfect steps than waiting for the perfect moment, where everything will hopefully lock in place. This rarely happens in life, so please take some action from today and commit to change your life! As the time goes by it will become effortless and part of who you are!

If you enjoyed this book, please spare a few minutes to write us a review. This way I will be aware of your opinion and feedback, so that I can provide more value to your lives.

Lastly, because I am a real cooking addict, I plan to launch a cookbook series with some very simple recipes, which everyone can make. If you are interested, visit this link and subscribe to our newsletter. You will be the first to be notified.
http://subscribe.theingeniouslifestyle.com/bonus

In addition, we are about to launch a coaching service, to help you apply the concepts in this book. Let's keep in touch through my website.
www.theingeniouslifestyle.com

Do not hesitate to contact me at :

chrispeters@theingeniouslifestyle.com

Wish you the best,

Chris Peters

Made in the USA
Lexington, KY
30 January 2017